Cupping Therapy Guide for Beginners

Understanding the Importance of Cupping Therapy

By

Archie Clayton

Table of Contents

CHAPTER 1

Introduction

1.1 What is Cupping Therapy

Cupping therapy, often simply referred to as "cupping," is a traditional alternative healing practice that has been employed for centuries in various cultures around the world. It involves the application of suction cups to the skin to create a vacuum seal, which draws the skin and underlying tissues upward into the cups. The resulting negative pressure can stimulate blood flow, relieve muscle tension, and promote overall relaxation and healing.

Cupping therapy is typically performed by trained practitioners who use specialized cups made of materials such as glass, silicone, or bamboo. These cups can be applied to specific points on the body, creating localized suction, or they can be moved across larger areas for a more dynamic effect. Cupping therapy is often used in conjunction with other traditional healing practices like acupuncture and massage.

1.2 History and Origins of Cupping Therapy

The history of cupping therapy is rich and diverse, with evidence of its use dating back thousands of years. It has been practiced in various forms across cultures including ancient Egyptian,

Chinese, Middle Eastern, and Greek civilizations.

- **Ancient China**: Cupping therapy has a particularly deep-rooted history in China, where it is believed to have originated over 2,000 years ago. In traditional Chinese medicine, cupping was used to balance the body's vital energy, known as "qi" or "chi," and to treat a wide range of ailments.

- **Ancient Egypt**: The ancient Egyptians also practiced cupping, with records dating back to 1550 BC. They used cupping as a means of treating fever, pain, and other illnesses.

- **Islamic Medicine**: In the Middle East, cupping therapy was embraced by Islamic medicine,

and it was described in early
medical texts. It became an
integral part of traditional Islamic
healing practices.

- **Hippocrates and Ancient
  Greece**: The famous Greek
  physician Hippocrates (c. 460-370
  BC) documented the use of
  cupping in ancient Greece. He
  recommended cupping for a
  variety of conditions, including
  menstrual problems and
  respiratory issues.

The widespread use of cupping
therapy across diverse cultures
suggests its enduring appeal and
potential therapeutic benefits.

1.3 Benefits and Purposes of Cupping Therapy

Cupping therapy offers a range of potential benefits and serves various purposes, which have contributed to its longevity as a healing practice:

- **Pain Relief**: Cupping can alleviate musculoskeletal pain, such as back pain, neck pain, and joint pain, by improving blood circulation and reducing muscle tension.

- **Improved Blood Flow**: By creating a vacuum seal on the skin, cupping can enhance blood circulation, which may help with the delivery of oxygen and nutrients to tissues and the removal of metabolic waste products.

- **Relaxation and Stress Reduction**: Many individuals find cupping therapy deeply relaxing and stress-relieving, making it an excellent complementary therapy for overall well-being.

- **Detoxification**: Some proponents suggest that cupping can aid in detoxification by drawing impurities and toxins to the surface of the skin, where they can be eliminated.

- **Respiratory Health**: Cupping is often used to address respiratory issues like colds, bronchitis, and asthma by promoting better lung function.

- **Digestive Health**: It can also be applied to alleviate digestive complaints and improve gastrointestinal function.

- **Skin Conditions**: Certain types of cupping, like wet cupping, may be used to treat skin conditions, such as acne and eczema.

1.4 Types of Cupping Therapy

Cupping therapy comes in various forms, each with its own techniques and applications:

- **Dry Cupping**: This is the most common form of cupping, where cups are placed on specific points on the body to create suction and stimulate blood flow and relaxation.

- **Wet Cupping**: Also known as "hijama" in Islamic medicine, this technique involves making small incisions on the skin before applying cups. It's believed to remove impurities and promote healing.

- **Fire Cupping**: In this traditional method, a flame is briefly introduced into the cup to create suction before applying it to the skin. It's often used in traditional Chinese medicine.

- **Silicone and Vacuum Cupping**: Modern variations of cupping use silicone cups and a vacuum pump to create suction, eliminating the need for flames.

- **Moving Cupping**: Cups are lubricated with oil and moved across the skin in a gliding motion. This technique is often used for muscle tension and pain relief.

cupping therapy is a time-tested holistic practice with a fascinating history, diverse benefits, and various techniques. Whether you're seeking pain relief, relaxation, or support for specific health conditions, understanding the fundamentals of cupping therapy can be a valuable step toward exploring its potential benefits for your well-being. It's important to consult with a qualified practitioner to ensure safe and effective cupping sessions.

CHAPTER 2

Tools and Equipment

2.1 Cups: Glass, Silicone, and Bamboo

Cups are a fundamental component of cupping therapy, and they come in different materials, each with its unique advantages and characteristics:

- **Glass Cups**: Glass cups are the traditional choice for cupping therapy. They are typically clear, allowing the therapist to monitor the skin's reaction during the session. Glass cups are often used in both stationary (dry) and moving (gliding) cupping techniques. Their smooth surface makes them easy to glide across the skin when applying moving cupping.

- **Silicone Cups**: Silicone cups have gained popularity in recent years due to their flexibility and ease of use. They are soft, pliable, and can be squeezed to create suction without the need for flames or pumps. Silicone cups are particularly well-suited for self-care and home use, as they are less intimidating and easier to handle than glass cups.

- **Bamboo Cups**: Bamboo cups are less common but have a niche following. They are usually handmade from bamboo and are known for their durability. Bamboo cups are often used in fire cupping, a traditional Chinese

technique involving the brief
introduction of flames to create
suction.

Each type of cup has its own
advantages, and the choice between
them often depends on the therapist's
preferences, the type of cupping being
performed, and the client's comfort
level.

2.2 Heat Sources: Fire Cupping vs. Vacuum Cupping

Heat sources are crucial in creating
the suction required for cupping
therapy. Two main methods are
employed:

- **Fire Cupping**: In traditional fire
  cupping, a flame is briefly

introduced into the cup to heat the air inside, creating a vacuum as the cup is quickly placed on the skin. The heat creates suction, and this method is often used for stationary cupping. Fire cupping requires skill and caution to ensure safety, and it is commonly seen in traditional Chinese medicine.

- **Vacuum Cupping**: Vacuum cupping uses mechanical devices to create suction without the need for an open flame. This method is often preferred for safety reasons and is commonly seen in modern cupping practices. It includes handheld pumps or electric suction machines that allow practitioners to control the level of suction more precisely.

The choice between fire cupping and vacuum cupping depends on the practitioner's training, the client's preferences, and the specific treatment goals.

2.3 Other Accessories

In addition to cups and heat sources, there are various accessories and tools that can be used in cupping therapy to enhance the experience and effectiveness of the treatment:

- **Massage Oil or Lotion**: Lubricating the skin with massage oil or lotion before applying cups makes it easier to glide them across the skin during moving cupping.

- **Alcohol or Cotton Balls**: These are used to clean the skin before cupping to reduce the risk of infection and to remove any oils or lotions that might interfere with suction.

- **Cupping Sets**: Cupping sets often include a variety of cup sizes and types, making them convenient for practitioners who need versatility in their treatments.

- **Cupping Sterilization Equipment**: Properly sterilizing cups and equipment is essential to ensure hygiene and prevent infections. Autoclaves or specialized sterilizers are used for this purpose.

- **Cupping Pump or Fire Torch**: These are used in conjunction with cups to create and regulate suction. In vacuum cupping, a pump is used, while fire cupping requires a torch to create the initial vacuum.

- **Cupping Marking Tools**: Some practitioners use marking tools like markers or specialized pens to mark specific points on the skin before cupping to aid in precise placement.

These accessories and tools play a significant role in ensuring the safety, effectiveness, and comfort of cupping therapy sessions. Experienced practitioners will often have a well-equipped setup tailored to their specific needs and the requirements of their clients.

CHAPTER 3

Preparing for Cupping Therapy

3.1 Safety Precautions

Safety should always be a top priority when preparing for cupping therapy. Both practitioners and clients should adhere to the following safety precautions:

- **Consultation and Assessment**: Before starting cupping therapy, practitioners should conduct a thorough consultation with the client. This includes discussing medical history, current health conditions, medications, and any specific concerns. Clients should provide honest and detailed information to ensure safe treatment.

- **Qualified Practitioner**: Seek out a qualified and licensed cupping therapist. They should have training in cupping techniques and a clear understanding of contraindications and safety measures.

- **Hygiene and Sterilization**: Ensure that all cups and equipment are properly cleaned and sterilized before each session. This minimizes the risk of infection. Single-use disposable cups are also an option for maximum hygiene.

- **Fire Safety**: If fire cupping is being performed, practitioners should be well-trained in the use of an open flame. Fire safety measures, such as a fire extinguisher and a fireproof surface, should be in place.

- **Allergies and Sensitivities**: Practitioners should be aware of any allergies or sensitivities that clients may have to materials used in cupping, such as oils, lotions, or specific cup materials.

- **Contraindications**: Both practitioners and clients should be familiar with contraindications, which are conditions or situations in which cupping therapy should not be used. Common contraindications include open wounds, sunburn, certain skin conditions, pregnancy, and severe medical conditions. When in doubt, consult with a healthcare provider.

- **Client Comfort**: Clients should communicate any discomfort or pain during the session, and practitioners should adjust suction or technique accordingly to ensure a comfortable experience.

3.2 Choosing the Right Location

Selecting the appropriate location for cupping therapy is essential for a safe and effective session:

- **Clean and Quiet Space**: Choose a clean and quiet space where both the practitioner and client can focus on the treatment without distractions.

- **Proper Lighting**: Ensure proper lighting to allow the practitioner to see the skin clearly and assess any reactions during the session.

- **Comfortable Temperature**: Maintain a comfortable room temperature to prevent discomfort during the therapy. Clients should be adequately covered to stay warm.

- **Treatment Table or Surface**: A padded treatment table or surface should be used to support the client's body during the session, ensuring comfort and stability.

- **Ventilation**: Adequate ventilation is important, especially if essential oils or any smoky methods like moxibustion are part of the treatment.

3.3 Skin Preparation

Skin preparation is a vital step to optimize the cupping experience and reduce the risk of complications:

- **Cleaning**: The skin in the treatment area should be thoroughly cleaned with mild soap and water to remove dirt, oils, and lotions. Afterward, it should be dried completely.

- **Hair Removal**: If the treatment area is particularly hairy, consider shaving or trimming the hair to ensure a proper seal between the cup and the skin.

- **Skin Sensitivity**: Assess the client's skin for any sensitivity or allergies to cupping materials or oils. Conduct a patch test if necessary.

- **Marking**: If specific points are being targeted, the practitioner may mark these points on the skin for precise cup placement.

following these preparation steps, both practitioners and clients can ensure that cupping therapy is conducted safely and effectively, enhancing the overall experience and therapeutic benefits of the treatment.

CHAPTER 4
Cupping Techniques

4.1 Dry Cupping

Dry cupping, also known as **stationary cupping**, is the most common and widely practiced form of cupping therapy. Here's a detailed explanation of this technique:

Procedure:

1. **Preparation**: The practitioner starts by selecting the appropriate cup size and material (usually glass, silicone, or bamboo) based on the treatment goals and the area of the body to be treated.

2. **Cleaning and Skin Preparation**: The treatment area on the client's skin is cleaned and, if necessary, lubricated with oil or lotion to facilitate the movement of cups.

3. **Application**: The cup is briefly heated using a flame (in fire cupping) or a mechanical pump (in vacuum cupping) to create suction. The practitioner then places the cup on the skin with the open end facing down, creating a vacuum seal. The skin is drawn upward into the cup due to the negative pressure inside.

4. **Suction Duration**: Depending on the client's tolerance and the practitioner's judgment, the cups can remain in place for a few minutes to up to 20

minutes. The duration can vary depending on the treatment objectives and the client's response.

5. **Removal**: To remove the cups, the practitioner typically releases the vacuum by pressing down on the skin near the edge of the cup or using a valve in the case of vacuum cups. The cups are then lifted away gently.

Benefits:

- **Pain Relief**: Dry cupping can provide relief from musculoskeletal pain and tension by promoting blood circulation and reducing muscle stiffness.

- **Relaxation**: Many clients find dry cupping deeply relaxing, making it beneficial for stress reduction and overall well-being.

- **Detoxification**: Some proponents suggest that dry cupping can help eliminate toxins and waste products from the body.

- **Improved Circulation**: By increasing blood flow to the treated area, dry cupping may enhance the delivery of oxygen and nutrients while aiding the removal of metabolic waste.

4.2 Wet Cupping

Wet cupping, also known as **hijama** in Islamic medicine, is a more involved form of cupping therapy that includes an additional step involving small incisions on the skin. Here's an overview of wet cupping:

Procedure:

1. **Initial Dry Cupping**: The process begins with dry cupping as described earlier. The practitioner selects the appropriate cups, creates suction, and applies them to the skin for a short period.

2. **Incisions**: After the initial dry cupping session, the practitioner removes the cups and makes small, superficial incisions (usually 3-4 small cuts) in the same area using a sterilized scalpel or lancet. These incisions are typically very shallow and painless.

3. **Second Cupping Session**: The same cups are then reapplied to

the area, drawing out a small amount of blood through the incisions and creating a vacuum seal.

4. **Suction Duration**: The cups are left in place for a few minutes to allow a small amount of blood to be collected into the cups.

5. **Removal and Care**: After the cups are removed, the practitioner cleans and disinfects the treated area, and sterile dressings may be applied to the incisions. Clients are advised to keep the area clean and avoid exposing it to water or excessive sweating for a period of time.

Benefits:

- **Detoxification**: Wet cupping is believed to promote detoxification by removing a small amount of stagnant blood and potentially harmful substances from the body.

- **Pain Relief**: Similar to dry cupping, wet cupping can provide pain relief by improving blood flow and reducing muscle tension.

- **Conditions Treated**: Wet cupping is often used to address specific health issues, such as migraines, respiratory problems, and hormonal imbalances.

It's important to note that wet cupping should only be performed by trained and qualified practitioners who follow strict hygiene and safety protocols.

Clients considering wet cupping should consult with a healthcare provider and ensure that they are suitable candidates for the procedure.

4.3 Flash Cupping

Flash cupping, also known as **flashfire cupping**, is a dynamic and stimulating form of cupping therapy. Unlike traditional stationary cupping, flash cupping involves brief and rapid application of cups with the use of fire. Here's how it works:

Procedure:

1. **Preparation**: The practitioner selects the appropriate cup size and material, typically glass cups, and prepares them for the treatment.

2. **Cleaning and Skin Preparation**: The treatment area on the client's skin is cleaned and sometimes lubricated with oil or lotion to facilitate movement.

3. **Fire Application**: Using a cotton ball soaked in alcohol, the practitioner ignites it and quickly places it inside the cup. The flame consumes the oxygen inside the cup, creating a vacuum as the cup is rapidly placed onto the client's skin. This creates an intense suction effect.

4. **Rapid Movement**: Flash cupping involves moving the cups across the skin while maintaining suction. The cups are typically moved in straight lines or specific patterns,

creating a strong pulling and
massaging sensation.

5. **Duration**: Flash cupping
   sessions are typically shorter
   than stationary cupping, usually
   lasting a few minutes.

6. **Removal**: After the session, the
   cups are removed by gently
   releasing the vacuum, and the
   treated area is assessed.

Benefits:

- **Stimulation**: Flash cupping
  provides a stimulating and
  invigorating experience. It is
  often used to address stagnant
  energy or blood circulation in
  the body.

- **Muscle Tension**: The rapid
  movement of cups can help
  alleviate muscle tension and

knots by stretching and relaxing the muscles.

- **Energizing Effect**: Some clients find flash cupping to be energizing and revitalizing due to its stimulating nature.

4.4 Moving Cupping

Moving cupping, also known as **gliding cupping**, is a cupping technique that involves continuous movement of cups across the skin. It combines the benefits of cupping with those of massage therapy, offering a dynamic and effective treatment. Here's how it's done:

Procedure:

1. **Preparation**: The practitioner selects the appropriate cups, often using silicone cups due to

their flexibility and ease of movement. They may also choose glass or bamboo cups for this technique.

2. **Cleaning and Skin Preparation**: The treatment area on the client's skin is cleaned and lubricated with massage oil or lotion to reduce friction and allow the cups to glide smoothly.

3. **Cup Placement**: Cups are applied to the skin, typically starting at one end of the area to be treated. The practitioner may use multiple cups to cover a larger area or target specific muscle groups.

4. **Movement**: With a gentle but firm grip, the practitioner moves the cups in a gliding

motion across the skin. The cups are kept in constant motion, creating a vacuum seal as they move.

5. **Technique Variation**: The practitioner can adjust the pressure and speed of cup movement based on the client's comfort level and treatment goals. They may focus on areas of tension or pain.

6. **Duration**: Moving cupping sessions can vary in duration, but they generally last longer than stationary cupping sessions, often ranging from 15 to 30 minutes.

7. **Removal**: After the session, the cups are removed, and the treated area is assessed for any

residual tension or changes in skin appearance.

Benefits:

- **Muscle Relaxation**: Moving cupping combines the benefits of cupping and massage, making it highly effective for relaxing tense muscles and relieving muscle knots.

- **Improved Circulation**: The continuous movement of cups enhances blood and lymphatic circulation, promoting the delivery of nutrients and removal of waste products.

- **Pain Relief**: This technique is often used to alleviate musculoskeletal pain and discomfort.

- **Stress Reduction**: Clients often find moving cupping to be deeply relaxing and a means of reducing stress and tension.

Both flash cupping and moving cupping are versatile techniques that can be tailored to the client's specific needs and preferences. They are typically performed by trained practitioners who can adjust the intensity and duration of treatment as required.

CHAPTER 5

The Cupping Process

5.1 Step-by-Step Instructions

A cupping therapy session generally follows a specific set of steps:

1. **Consultation and Assessment**: The session often begins with a consultation between the practitioner and the client. During this discussion, the client's medical history, current health conditions, and treatment goals are reviewed. The practitioner assesses whether cupping is suitable for the client and identifies the areas to be treated.

2. **Preparation**: The treatment room is set up with the necessary equipment, including the cups, heat source (if applicable), massage oil or lotion, and any other accessories. The client is positioned comfortably on a treatment table or surface.

3. **Cleaning and Skin Preparation**: The skin in the area to be treated is cleaned with mild soap and water to remove dirt, oils, and lotions. After cleaning, the skin is dried thoroughly.

4. **Cup Selection**: The practitioner selects the appropriate type and size of cups based on the treatment goals and the client's needs. Glass, silicone, or bamboo cups may be chosen.

5. **Suction Application**: The cups are prepared for suction. For fire cupping, a flame is briefly introduced into the cup to create a vacuum, and then the cup is placed on the skin. In vacuum cupping, a mechanical pump or electric suction machine is used to create the vacuum. The cups are applied to the skin, and a vacuum seal is formed, drawing the skin upward into the cups.

6. **Suction Duration**: The cups remain in place for a predetermined duration. The length of time can vary from a few minutes to up to 20 minutes, depending on the treatment plan, the client's comfort level, and the practitioner's assessment.

7. **Monitoring**: Throughout the session, the practitioner monitors

the client's skin for any adverse reactions, such as excessive redness or discomfort. Adjustments to the cups may be made if necessary to ensure the client's comfort.

8. **Removal**: At the end of the session, the cups are removed. For stationary cupping, the practitioner gently releases the vacuum seal by pressing down on the skin near the edge of the cups. In the case of vacuum cups, a valve is often used to release the suction. Cups are lifted away gently and placed aside.

9. **Aftercare**: After cupping, the treated area may be assessed, and the practitioner may recommend specific aftercare instructions. This may include avoiding exposure to cold or wind, staying hydrated, and

refraining from strenuous physical activity for a period.

10. **Consultation and Follow-up**: The practitioner may conduct a brief post-session consultation with the client to discuss the treatment's effects and any recommendations for follow-up sessions or additional therapies.

5.2 Duration and Frequency

The duration and frequency of cupping therapy sessions can vary depending on the client's needs and the practitioner's recommendations. Here are some general guidelines:

- **Duration**: A single cupping session typically lasts between 15 minutes to 1 hour, with the average

duration being around 30 minutes.
The length of the session can be
adjusted based on the client's
comfort and treatment objectives.

- **Frequency**: The frequency of
  cupping sessions can vary widely.
  For some acute issues, such as
  muscle tension or pain, clients may
  benefit from more frequent
  sessions, such as once or twice a
  week. For chronic conditions or
  maintenance of overall well-being,
  less frequent sessions, such as
  once a month, may be appropriate.

- **Individualized Approach**: The
  ideal frequency and duration of
  cupping therapy should be
  determined on an individual basis.
  It depends on factors like the
  client's health goals, the specific
  condition being treated, and how
  the client responds to the therapy.

Consultation with a qualified cupping practitioner is essential to develop a personalized treatment plan.

It's important to note that cupping therapy is generally considered safe when performed by trained professionals who follow hygiene and safety protocols. However, clients should communicate openly with their practitioners about their comfort level and any concerns during and after the sessions to ensure a positive and effective experience.

5.3 Sensations During Cupping

During a cupping therapy session, clients may experience various sensations, some of which are quite common and expected. These sensations can provide insight into the effectiveness of the treatment and the body's response to cupping. Here are the sensations that clients might encounter during cupping therapy:

1. **Suction and Pressure**: The initial sensation when the cups are applied is the feeling of suction and pressure on the skin. Depending on the strength of the suction, this can range from mild to moderate pressure.

2. **Tingling and Warmth**: Many clients report a tingling or warming sensation in and around the area where the cups are placed. This is often attributed to increased blood circulation as the cups draw blood toward the surface of the skin.

3. **Tightness or Tugging**: As the skin
    is drawn upward into the cups,
    clients may feel a sensation of
    tightness or tugging. This can be
    especially noticeable when the
    cups are first applied.

4. **Heat**: In fire cupping, clients may
    experience a mild sensation of
    warmth as the practitioner briefly
    introduces a flame into the cup
    before applying it to the skin.

5. **Mild Discomfort**: Some clients
    may experience mild discomfort or
    a sense of pressure during the
    session, especially if the cups are
    placed on areas with underlying
    muscle tension or knots.

6. **Relaxation**: On the flip side, many
    clients find cupping therapy deeply
    relaxing. As the cups promote
    blood flow and release muscle

tension, they may experience a sense of calm and relaxation.

7. **Itching or Tickling**: Occasionally, clients may report mild itching or tickling sensations in the treated area. This is typically temporary and can be attributed to increased blood flow and nerve stimulation.

8. **Pain Relief**: One of the primary goals of cupping therapy is to provide pain relief. Many clients experience a reduction in pain and discomfort during or after the session.

9. **Bruising and Discoloration**: After cupping, it's common to observe circular marks on the skin, which can range from pink to deep purple. These marks, known as "cupping marks" or "cupping bruises," are a result of the suction

and are not typically painful. They
usually fade within a few days to a
couple of weeks.

10. **Energizing or Invigorating**:
Some clients report feeling
energized or invigorated after a
cupping session, attributing this
sensation to improved circulation
and the release of muscle tension.

It's important to note that the intensity
of these sensations can vary from
person to person and can depend on
factors like the type of cupping
technique used, the strength of
suction, and the client's individual
sensitivity. Communication with the
cupping practitioner is key during the
session. Clients should feel
comfortable discussing any sensations
they experience, especially if they are

concerned or uncomfortable. Practitioners can adjust the cups or the technique as needed to ensure a positive and effective experience.

CHAPTER 6

Aftercare and Recovery

After a cupping therapy session, proper aftercare is essential to optimize the benefits of the treatment and minimize any potential side effects. Here are guidelines for post-cupping care:

6.1 Post-Cupping Care

1. **Hydration**: Drink plenty of water after your cupping session. Proper hydration helps the body flush out toxins that may have been released during the treatment. Staying well-hydrated is important in the hours

and days following cupping therapy.

2. **Rest and Relaxation**: It's advisable to take it easy after a cupping session, especially if you had a vigorous or intense treatment. Rest and relaxation can help your body recover and maximize the therapeutic effects of cupping.

3. **Avoid Exposure to Cold or Wind**: After cupping, your skin may be more sensitive. To prevent discomfort, avoid exposure to cold temperatures, strong winds, or drafts. Dress warmly and protect the treated areas from chill.

4. **Avoid Strenuous Activity**: Refrain from strenuous physical activities, heavy workouts, or intense exercise for at least 24

hours after cupping. Give your body time to recover and avoid overexertion.

5. **Avoid Hot Showers or Baths**: While your skin may feel warm after cupping, it's best to avoid hot showers or baths immediately after the session. Lukewarm water is generally recommended. This helps prevent overheating and excessive sweating, which can irritate the skin.

6. **Avoid Alcohol and Caffeine**: For the remainder of the day after cupping, it's a good idea to avoid alcohol and caffeine, as these substances can potentially disrupt the body's ability to detoxify and heal.

7. **Monitor Your Skin**: Check the treated areas for any signs of

irritation, redness, or bruising. It's normal to see circular marks on the skin (cupping marks) that may range from pink to deep purple. These marks typically fade within a few days to a couple of weeks and are not typically painful. If you notice any unusual skin reactions or discomfort, contact your cupping practitioner.

8. **Moisturize**: If your skin feels dry or irritated after cupping, consider applying a gentle, hypoallergenic moisturizer to keep it hydrated. Avoid heavy or scented lotions that might irritate the skin.

9. **Avoid Sun Exposure**: Protect the cupped areas from direct sun exposure, especially if they are sensitive or have cupping marks. Sunscreen or clothing that covers

the skin can help prevent further
irritation.

10. **Consult Your Practitioner**: If
you have any concerns or
questions about your post-cupping
care, don't hesitate to reach out to
your cupping therapist. They can
provide guidance and address any
specific issues you may encounter.

Individual experiences with cupping
therapy can vary. Some clients may
feel immediate relief and energized,
while others may initially experience
mild discomfort or fatigue. These
reactions are often temporary and part
of the body's natural healing process.
If you're new to cupping, it's a good
practice to discuss your post-
treatment sensations and any
questions you have with your
practitioner during your session or
follow-up consultations. This helps

ensure that you have a positive and beneficial cupping experience.

6.2 Common Side Effects

Cupping therapy is generally safe when performed by trained professionals who follow hygiene and safety protocols. However, like any therapeutic treatment, there can be side effects or reactions. Here are common side effects associated with cupping and guidelines for when to seek medical advice:

1. **Cupping Marks**: One of the most common side effects of cupping therapy is the appearance of circular marks on the skin. These marks, often referred to as "cupping marks" or "cupping bruises," can range from pink to deep purple. They are caused by

the suction of the cups and are not typically painful. Cupping marks usually fade within a few days to a couple of weeks.

2. **Temporary Skin Discoloration**: In addition to cupping marks, the treated skin area may appear red, pink, or slightly discolored immediately after the session. This discoloration is usually temporary and resolves within a short time.

3. **Skin Sensitivity**: Some clients may experience mild skin sensitivity or tenderness in the treated area, particularly if the cups were applied with strong suction or if multiple cups were used in one area.

4. **Itching or Tingling**: Itching or tingling sensations on or around the cupped areas are relatively

common and can be attributed to increased blood circulation and nerve stimulation. These sensations are typically mild and temporary.

5. **Fatigue or Lightheadedness**: After a cupping session, some clients may feel temporarily fatigued or lightheaded. This is often due to the relaxation induced by the therapy and is usually short-lived.

6. **Slight Swelling**: In some cases, the skin in the cupped area may appear slightly swollen or puffy immediately after the session. This is generally a transient reaction and should subside on its own.

6.3 When to Seek Medical Advice

While cupping therapy is generally safe, there are situations where it's advisable to seek medical advice or attention:

1. **Severe Pain**: If you experience severe or persistent pain during or after cupping therapy, it's essential to consult with a healthcare provider. Severe pain may indicate an issue that requires medical evaluation.

2. **Severe Skin Reactions**: While cupping marks are common and typically harmless, if you notice severe skin reactions, such as excessive blistering, open sores, or signs of infection (e.g., redness, swelling, warmth, or pus), seek medical attention promptly.

3. **Allergic Reactions**: If you develop an allergic reaction to any substances used during cupping, such as oils, lotions, or cup materials, consult with a healthcare provider. Allergic reactions can manifest as itching, rash, hives, or difficulty breathing and require prompt attention.

4. **Persistent Discomfort**: If you experience prolonged discomfort, itching, or skin sensitivity that doesn't improve or worsens over time, it's advisable to consult with a healthcare provider or your cupping practitioner.

5. **Unusual Symptoms**: If you notice any unusual or concerning symptoms that you believe may be related to cupping therapy, don't hesitate to seek medical advice. This includes symptoms like

dizziness, nausea, or shortness of breath that may not be typical reactions.

6. **Preexisting Medical Conditions**: If you have preexisting medical conditions, especially those related to blood clotting disorders or skin disorders, consult with your healthcare provider before undergoing cupping therapy to ensure it is safe and appropriate for you.

Effective communication with your cupping practitioner is vital. If you experience any discomfort or have concerns during or after a cupping session, it's advisable to discuss these issues with your practitioner. They can provide guidance, adjust their techniques, or address any specific concerns you may have. Additionally, if you have any doubts or questions about the safety and suitability of cupping for your individual circumstances, consult with a qualified healthcare professional.

CHAPTER 7

Conditions Treated with Cupping Therapy

Cupping therapy is a versatile treatment that can be used to address a wide range of health conditions and concerns. Here, we'll explore the categories of conditions that are often treated with cupping therapy:

7.1 Pain Management

Cupping therapy is frequently employed as a complementary or alternative approach to manage various types of pain, both acute and chronic. It can be effective in providing relief from the following pain-related conditions:

- **Musculoskeletal Pain**: Cupping is often used to alleviate muscle tension, stiffness, and pain. It can be particularly helpful for conditions such as back pain, neck pain, shoulder pain, and muscle knots.

- **Arthritis**: People with arthritis, including osteoarthritis and rheumatoid arthritis, may find relief from joint pain and stiffness through cupping therapy.

- **Headaches and Migraines**: Cupping applied to the neck, shoulders, and upper back can help relieve tension headaches and migraines by improving blood flow and relaxing tense muscles.

- **Sports Injuries**: Athletes often turn to cupping therapy to address sports-related injuries like sprains, strains, and overuse injuries. It can promote healing and reduce pain and inflammation.

- **Fibromyalgia**: Cupping therapy may provide relief for some individuals with fibromyalgia by reducing muscle pain and promoting relaxation.

- **Menstrual Pain**: Some women use cupping to manage menstrual cramps and associated lower abdominal pain.

7.2 Respiratory Issues

Cupping therapy can be employed as an adjunctive therapy for various respiratory conditions. It aims to improve lung function, clear congestion, and reduce inflammation. Common respiratory issues treated with cupping include:

- **Asthma**: Cupping therapy is used to alleviate asthma symptoms by promoting relaxation of respiratory muscles, reducing bronchial inflammation, and helping to clear mucus from the airways.

- **Bronchitis**: For acute bronchitis, cupping can aid in loosening mucus and relieving chest congestion, making it easier for the body to expel phlegm.

- **Cough and Cold**: Cupping applied to the upper back can be used as a part of cold and flu relief strategies to reduce chest congestion and ease coughing.

- **Chronic Obstructive Pulmonary Disease (COPD)**: Some individuals with COPD may use cupping therapy to improve lung function and reduce symptoms such as shortness of breath.

- **Allergic Rhinitis**: Cupping on the upper back and shoulders may help alleviate symptoms of allergic rhinitis by reducing inflammation and promoting sinus drainage.

It's important to note that while cupping therapy can be beneficial for managing pain and respiratory issues, it should not replace conventional medical treatments or medications prescribed by healthcare providers. Cupping is often used in conjunction with other therapies as part of a comprehensive treatment plan. Before considering cupping therapy for any medical condition, it's advisable to consult with a qualified healthcare professional to ensure it is appropriate and safe for your specific needs and circumstances. Additionally, cupping should only be performed by trained and qualified practitioners who adhere to hygiene and safety standards.

7.3 Digestive Problems

Cupping therapy can potentially benefit individuals with various digestive issues by promoting relaxation, improving blood flow, and stimulating the body's natural healing processes. Some of the digestive problems that may be addressed with cupping include:

- **Indigestion**: Cupping therapy can be applied to the abdomen to promote relaxation of digestive muscles and enhance blood circulation in the abdominal area, potentially aiding in digestion and reducing symptoms of indigestion.

- **Constipation**: Cupping may help alleviate constipation by promoting relaxation and reducing tension in the abdominal muscles. This can encourage bowel movements and relieve discomfort.

- **Irritable Bowel Syndrome (IBS)**: While cupping therapy is not a direct treatment for IBS, it can be used to manage stress and anxiety, which are known triggers for IBS symptoms. Reducing stress through cupping may lead to symptom improvement.

- **Bloating**: Cupping applied to the abdominal region may help relieve bloating by improving circulation and reducing tension in the abdominal muscles.

- **Nausea**: In some cases, cupping on the upper back or shoulders can promote relaxation and alleviate nausea. It is often used in conjunction with other approaches for nausea relief.

It's important to note that cupping therapy for digestive problems is often used as a complementary approach alongside dietary and lifestyle changes, as well as conventional medical treatments when necessary. Consulting with a healthcare provider or a qualified cupping therapist is advisable to determine the suitability of cupping for your specific digestive issues.

7.4 Skin Conditions

Cupping therapy can have applications in managing various skin conditions. While cupping is not a primary treatment for skin disorders, it can promote skin health and help address certain issues. Some skin conditions where cupping may be considered include:

- **Acne**: Facial cupping, when performed gently and with appropriate oils or serums, can help improve blood circulation, lymphatic drainage, and the absorption of skincare products. It may aid in reducing acne inflammation and promoting healthier skin.

- **Eczema**: For individuals with eczema, cupping therapy can help with symptom management by

reducing itching and inflammation.
However, it should be performed
with caution to avoid exacerbating
skin irritation.

- **Cellulite**: Body cupping is
  sometimes used as a part of
  cellulite reduction treatments. It is
  believed to improve blood flow,
  reduce fluid retention, and
  temporarily improve the
  appearance of cellulite.

- **Psoriasis**: Cupping may help
  alleviate some of the discomfort
  associated with psoriasis, such as
  itching and inflammation. Again, it
  should be performed gently to
  avoid aggravating the condition.

- **Scarring**: Cupping therapy can
  promote blood circulation and
  collagen production, potentially
  aiding in the healing of scars. It is

sometimes used alongside other scar management techniques.

For skin-related concerns, it's important to consult with a qualified dermatologist or skincare specialist to determine the best treatment plan for your specific condition. Cupping therapy, if used, should be performed by a trained and experienced practitioner who is knowledgeable about skincare and skin conditions to avoid any adverse effects.

Always remember that cupping therapy should be integrated into a comprehensive healthcare plan and should not replace medical treatments prescribed by healthcare professionals for digestive problems or skin conditions.

7.5 Emotional Well-being

Cupping therapy can have a positive impact on emotional well-being by promoting relaxation, reducing stress, and creating a sense of overall balance and wellness. While cupping is not a replacement for mental health treatments, it can be a valuable complementary approach to support emotional well-being. Here's how cupping can benefit emotional health:

1. Stress Reduction: Cupping therapy induces deep relaxation by stimulating the parasympathetic nervous system, which counters the body's stress response. This relaxation can help reduce feelings of tension, anxiety, and stress.

2. Improved Sleep: Many individuals find that cupping therapy helps improve the quality of their sleep. Better sleep can lead to improved mood and a greater sense of emotional well-being.

3. Muscle Relaxation: Cupping can alleviate muscle tension and knots, which are often physical manifestations of stress. By reducing muscle tension, cupping can help individuals feel more relaxed and comfortable.

4. Enhanced Circulation: Improved blood circulation and lymphatic drainage resulting from cupping can enhance the delivery of oxygen and nutrients to the body's cells, potentially leading to increased energy levels and a more positive outlook.

5. Mind-Body Connection: The physical sensation of cupping can foster a stronger connection between the mind and body, promoting mindfulness and self-awareness. This heightened awareness can contribute to emotional well-being.

6. Holistic Wellness: Cupping is often viewed as a holistic wellness practice, and many individuals find that incorporating holistic approaches into their self-care routines enhances their emotional well-being.

It's important to approach cupping therapy as one component of a comprehensive approach to emotional well-being. Combining cupping with other practices like meditation, exercise, and counseling can provide a more holistic approach to maintaining mental health.

If you are experiencing emotional difficulties, stress, or mental health challenges, it's essential to seek support from a qualified mental health professional or counselor. While cupping can be a helpful addition to your self-care routine, it should not replace professional mental health treatment when needed. A qualified healthcare provider can assess your specific needs and provide guidance on the most appropriate treatment options to support your emotional well-being.

CHAPTER 8

Cupping Therapy Myths and Misconceptions

Cupping therapy, like many alternative and complementary treatments, has its fair share of myths and misconceptions. Here we'll debunk some common myths and address safety concerns related to cupping therapy.

8.1 Debunking Common Myths

Myth 1: Cupping therapy is painful.

- Debunked: While cupping can cause sensations like suction and pressure, it is generally not painful. Most people describe the sensation as unique but not painful. If you experience significant pain during a cupping session, it's important to communicate this with your practitioner as they can adjust the treatment to ensure your comfort.

Myth 2: Cupping therapy leaves permanent scars.

- Debunked: Cupping marks, which can resemble bruises, are a common side effect of cupping. However, they are temporary and typically fade within a few days to a couple of weeks. Permanent scarring from cupping is extremely rare.

Myth 3: Cupping therapy removes toxins from the body.

- Debunked: Cupping is often associated with detoxification, but the scientific basis for this claim is limited. While cupping can promote circulation and potentially stimulate the lymphatic system, the idea that it removes specific toxins from the body remains unproven.

Myth 4: Cupping therapy can cure or treat all diseases.

- Debunked: Cupping is not a
  panacea and cannot cure or
  treat all diseases. It is most
  commonly used as a
  complementary therapy to
  manage certain conditions and
  alleviate symptoms. It should
  not be relied upon as a sole
  treatment for serious medical
  conditions.

Myth 5: Cupping therapy is unregulated and unsafe.

- Debunked: Cupping therapy is
  regulated in many countries,
  and professional cupping
  practitioners often undergo
  training and certification. When
  performed by trained and
  qualified practitioners who
  follow hygiene and safety
  protocols, cupping therapy is
  generally considered safe.

8.2 Safety Concerns

While cupping therapy is generally safe when performed correctly, there are some safety concerns to be aware of:

1. **Bruising and Skin Sensitivity**: Cupping can cause temporary bruising and skin sensitivity. It's important to ensure that the cups are applied at the appropriate level of suction to minimize these side effects. If you have a bleeding disorder or are taking blood-thinning medications, consult your healthcare provider before undergoing cupping.

2. **Infection Risk**: If the cups or equipment are not properly cleaned and sterilized, there is a risk of infection. Always seek

cupping therapy from a reputable practitioner who follows strict hygiene practices.

3. **Burns**: Fire cupping, which involves briefly introducing a flame into the cup, carries a risk of burns if not performed correctly. Practitioners should be skilled in fire cupping techniques to minimize this risk.

4. **Allergic Reactions**: Some individuals may be allergic to the oils, lotions, or materials used during cupping therapy. If you have known allergies or sensitivities, inform your practitioner beforehand.

5. **Misuse or Overuse**: Overuse of cupping therapy or excessive suction can lead to skin damage or discomfort. It's important to work

with a qualified practitioner who can tailor the treatment to your specific needs.

6. **Preexisting Health Conditions**: Individuals with certain medical conditions, such as hemophilia, skin infections, or open wounds, should avoid cupping or seek guidance from a healthcare provider before undergoing treatment.

7. **Pregnancy and Certain Medical Conditions**: Pregnant individuals and those with certain medical conditions (e.g., cancer, deep vein thrombosis, organ failure) should consult with their healthcare provider before considering cupping therapy, as it may not be suitable for all circumstances.

To ensure a safe cupping experience, it's essential to choose a qualified and experienced practitioner who follows safety guidelines and uses sterile equipment. Communication with your practitioner about your medical history, allergies, and any concerns is also crucial for a safe and effective treatment.

CHAPTER 9

Combining Cupping Therapy with Other Practices

Cupping therapy can be effectively combined with various other complementary practices to enhance its therapeutic benefits. Two common combinations are cupping and acupuncture, as well as cupping and massage. Let's explore how these integrative approaches work:

9.1 Cupping and Acupuncture

Cupping and acupuncture are often used together in a complementary approach known as "acupuncture cupping" or "acu-cupping." These therapies share some common principles and can synergize to provide comprehensive health benefits. Here's how they work together:

1. **Acupuncture**: Acupuncture involves the insertion of thin needles into specific acupuncture points on the body to stimulate energy flow (Qi) and promote healing. It is used to address a wide range of health issues, including pain, stress, and various medical conditions.

2. **Cupping**: Cupping therapy creates suction on the skin's surface to increase blood flow, relax muscles, and promote healing. It can be used to address pain, muscle tension, and certain health conditions.

3. **Combination**: Acupuncturists often incorporate cupping into their treatments. This can involve placing cups on specific acupuncture points or using cupping as a precursor to acupuncture. Cupping can help prepare the body by improving circulation and relaxing muscles, making acupuncture more effective.

4. **Enhanced Blood Flow**: Both cupping and acupuncture promote improved blood circulation. Cupping helps draw blood to the

surface, while acupuncture needles stimulate blood flow within the body. Enhanced circulation can support the delivery of nutrients and oxygen to cells and tissues, aiding in the body's natural healing processes.

5. **Pain Relief**: The combination of cupping and acupuncture is particularly effective for pain management. Cupping can alleviate muscle tension and knots, while acupuncture can target specific pain points and provide pain relief.

6. **Stress Reduction**: Acupuncture is known for its stress-reducing effects by promoting relaxation and reducing anxiety. When combined with cupping, this relaxation effect can be enhanced,

providing emotional well-being benefits.

7. **Holistic Approach**: The integration of cupping and acupuncture allows for a holistic approach to health and wellness. By addressing both physical and energetic aspects of the body, individuals can experience comprehensive healing benefits.

9.2 Cupping and Massage

Cupping and massage are another complementary combination that offers a unique and comprehensive therapeutic experience. Here's how they work together:

1. **Massage**: Massage therapy involves manual manipulation of

soft tissues to relieve muscle tension, reduce stress, and promote relaxation. It is known for its benefits in alleviating musculoskeletal pain and promoting overall well-being.

2. **Cupping**: Cupping therapy can be used in conjunction with massage. Cups are applied to the skin, and the practitioner uses gliding or stationary cupping techniques over the oiled or lotioned skin. This combines the benefits of cupping and massage into a single treatment.

3. **Enhanced Muscle Relaxation**: The combination of massage and cupping enhances muscle relaxation. The suction effect of cupping can help release muscle tension and knots, making it easier

for the massage therapist to work on problem areas.

4. **Improved Circulation**: Both cupping and massage promote improved blood and lymphatic circulation. This can enhance the delivery of oxygen and nutrients to muscle tissues and aid in the removal of waste products, promoting faster recovery.

5. **Pain Relief**: The joint effects of massage and cupping can provide effective pain relief. This is particularly beneficial for individuals with chronic pain conditions, such as back pain or tension headaches.

6. **Stress Reduction**: Massage therapy is renowned for its stress-reducing properties. When combined with cupping, clients

often experience a deeper sense of relaxation and stress relief.

7. **Detoxification**: Some proponents believe that the combination of cupping and massage can assist in the detoxification process by promoting the removal of metabolic waste and toxins from the body.

When considering cupping therapy in combination with acupuncture or massage, it's essential to seek qualified practitioners who are experienced in these integrated approaches. Effective communication with your practitioners is also crucial to ensure that the combination of therapies aligns with your specific health goals and needs.

9.3 Cupping and Traditional Chinese Medicine

Cupping therapy has deep historical and philosophical roots in **Traditional Chinese Medicine (TCM)**, and it is often used as an integral part of TCM practices. Here's how cupping and TCM work together:

1. **TCM Principles**: Cupping therapy aligns with key TCM principles, including the concept of Qi (pronounced "chee"), meridians, and the balance of Yin and Yang. According to TCM, when Qi flow is disrupted or blocked along meridians, health issues can arise. Cupping is used to restore the free flow of Qi and balance the body's energy.

2. **Meridian-Based Treatment**: In TCM, specific acupuncture points on the body correspond to different organs and systems. Cupping can be used in a meridian-based approach, with cups placed on or moved along specific acupuncture points to address imbalances or health concerns associated with those points.

3. **Qi and Blood Flow**: Cupping is believed to promote the movement of Qi and blood in the body. It is used to alleviate stagnation, which is considered a common cause of various health problems in TCM. By enhancing the circulation of Qi and blood, cupping can support the body's natural healing processes.

4. **Balance of Yin and Yang**: TCM emphasizes the balance of Yin (negative, cooling, and passive)

and Yang (positive, heating, and active) energies within the body. Cupping is used to restore this balance by either clearing excessive heat (Yang) or nourishing Yin deficiencies, depending on the individual's TCM diagnosis.

5. **Detoxification**: Cupping is sometimes employed in TCM as a method to promote detoxification and the elimination of pathogenic factors. It is believed to draw out toxins and excess heat from the body.

6. **Pain Management**: TCM often views pain as a result of Qi and blood stagnation. Cupping therapy can be a valuable component of TCM pain management strategies. It is used to relieve muscle tension

and discomfort by promoting the free flow of Qi and blood.

7. **Holistic Approach**: TCM takes a holistic approach to health and wellness, considering the interconnectedness of body, mind, and spirit. Cupping aligns with this holistic perspective, as it addresses both physical and energetic aspects of health.

8. **Individualized Treatment**: In TCM, treatment plans are highly individualized based on the patient's unique constitution and patterns of disharmony. Cupping is adapted to each individual's specific TCM diagnosis and health goals.

9. **Herbal Medicine Integration**: In some cases, cupping therapy is combined with herbal medicine in

TCM. Herbal formulas may be prescribed to support and enhance the effects of cupping treatment.

Overall, cupping therapy and TCM complement each other by addressing the body's energetic and physical aspects. When seeking cupping therapy within a TCM context, it is advisable to consult with a qualified TCM practitioner who has a deep understanding of both cupping and traditional Chinese medical principles. This ensures that the treatment aligns with your individual health needs and follows the holistic approach of TCM.